No More MS

by

Deborah Lynn Lovell

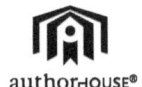

authorHOUSE®

AuthorHouse™
1663 Liberty Drive, Suite 200
Bloomington, IN 47403
www.authorhouse.com
Phone: 1-800-839-8640

First published by AuthorHouse   10/18/2007

ISBN: 978-1-4343-4390-1 (sc)

Printed in the United States of America
Bloomington, Indiana

This book is printed on acid-free paper.

Special Dedication

This book is dedicated to my mom, Joyce Rodriguez. I couldn't have gotten through this painful experience without her love and support. It really is a miracle on how her support, understanding was used to love me at the highest level any human being could accomplished at such a painful time. This sickness that hit my body wasn't only physical it was emotional and spiritual.

The letter on the following pages will give you a short understanding of my pain when attacked with multiple sclerosis. My background from the upbringing in Brooklyn, New York, the move to Fayetteville, Georgia and Ministry School training in Southfield, Michigan all played a part in my fight against multiple sclerosis.

There is no other mom, like mine. I wouldn't be here before or after the attack of MS had she not been the mom that wears the 1,000 different hats that it took to handle my pain.

The letter on the following pages was distributed to various family members, friends and/or associates that poured their love and support in me for three years straight.

Deborah Lovell's Testimony
(2003-2006)

Hey Everyone:

I just wanted to give a love shout to everyone. Of course, I have a lot to say; don't act like you don't know me by now-->smile.

For your information, none of what I speak about has anything to do with my Ministry training, or Religion. It has everything to do with my love for God and His people. Please ask my mom, I have been helping groups of people since the age of 13. You all know where I got if from-->smile mom.

Anyhow, November 2006 will be three years since my mom had to come get me out of Michigan because my body broke down from MS and I was in denial and couldn't believe MS had the nerve to attack me; most of you know the story.

I was in pretty bad shape when getting off the plan: 1. Starting losing memory quickly; 2.Could not physically groom myself from brushing my teeth to combing my hair; 3. Walking was almost impossible; 4. Pain unbearable; 5.Spiritually and Emotionally broken; 6.Talking with some volume wasn't there; 7.Depressed and not forgiving/loving attitude.

It has really been my family that did the kick-off and the friends and or divine associates for that time followed up. Just to give you some of the curing medicine received. My mother never left my side for 2 years; my sister kept the house going with food, support and love. My daughter literally trained me on how I trained her; she was not having me feeling sorry for myself especially as I got better; can you believe that I am the mother not her.

12 people from my church called me everyday for one year; even 2 from Michigan, visitors from all over came to love and encourage me. I have no idea where these folks are today. When able people came and took me to Church, lunches, dinners, overnights and 2 trips to Florida this went on for almost 2 years straight.-->God is good all the time.

Although there have been ups and downs my faith in God's love for me, the best family and the greatest friends have carried me and to be honest I couldn't have gotten through without them especially my family.

At the present time, there have been challenges but look how far we have come. Thanksgiving this year will be very special to me. In addition to feeling better, my insides were getting cleaned up as well. Did you know I had the nerve to be prideful? and more but being home and allowing God to show me I live in His World, He doesn't live in mine showed me a thing or two. Lesson # 1, 1501 is now in session, Ministry School cannot compare to Private courses.

I hope you will rejoice with me this Holiday Season in giving God thanks for sending the world to help me so when I truly recover all will say that was "God".

Love you all,

Sincerely,

Deborah Lynn Lovell

No More MS

Do you have multiple sclerosis (MS) or multiple scars? It is only after I was diagnosed with MS that I learned how many emotional scars were hidden in my heart, such as un-forgiveness, a judgmental attitude, and some character flaws. Before I begin there are other simlinaries that I believe many MS patients have in common, such as:

- ◆ A-type personalities (workaholics)
- ◆ Emotional hidden behavior patterns
- ◆ Poor eating habits
- ◆ Longtime absence from children
- ◆ Pneumonia

All the above behavior problems may have added to the MS systems. To inform those of you who don't know about or have no experience with A-type personalities, they are the most helpful and compassionate people when it comes to their jobs, projects, or certain people but they never treat themselves with that same respect (I Cor. 6:19-20). The word *vacation* is not in their vocabulary.

To tell you the truth, my emotional pain was held in and that caused more damage to my body than anything else. Although you couldn't see my pain outside, my actions would show, such as a working schedule that no human being could keep up with. The drinks of coffee and soda, and sugar, along with hamburgers, were my lifeline to a food supply.

My daughter is twenty-four years of age (2004), at the time of this writing. There has not been a baby in our family for almost twenty-five years. I mention that because some studies show MS patients haven't had children in their presence for years at a time.

I had pneumonia twice back to back in 1999 and 2000, and that still did not slow me down. The moment I got out of the hospital, work was what I ran to.

My desire to love people in an unbalanced fashion could have cost me my life.

A questionnaire will be listed at the end of this book. It will determine if you have the emotional part of MS (multiple scars) that can kill you mentally. If not, praise God and continue being obedient. If yes, please see some of the suggestions.

Before I begin this story, let me tell you one of the major affects that hurts people dealing with multiple sclerosis; that is stress. My whole life has been centered on dealing with high levels of stressful situations. I started off with my daughter's dad. I had dated him fifteen years and then he broke my heart.

I really didn't pay any attention to myself. It was always about other people. My health was something I took for granted and paid no attention to. It was only after being attacked by this disease that I noted behavior patterns had a lot to do with my upbringing.

Remember MS and stress doesn't mix. I am going to list a few items that happened during this time and you tell me how in the world this book has been able to be written and you are able to understand. Let me also give you some information about MS before the listed stress items.

> **Multiple Sclerosis**: Most researchers believe MS is an "autoimmune disease" – one in which white blood cells, meant to fight infection or disease, are misguided to target and attack the body's own cells. This attack causes inflammation in the Central Nervous System (CNS), which may damage the myelin and ultimately injure the nerves. This information was gathered from: "The Multiple Sclerosis Association of America" - All About Multiple Sclerosis, Third Edition, MSAA.

Some of the systems I had included:
1. Not able to comprehend conversations
2. Creating offensive behavior yet you are unaware
3. Speaking what you are thinking out loud

There are many other behavior patterns that occur with this disease. What had happened with me is that to a certain extent I really was doing well when I got home from living in Michigan, but some stressful situations occurred and the hurt almost sent me toward death again. But, praise God, many of the people whom He surrounded me with were Christian folks and they were able to minister to me.

There is a ministry that most people don't want to touch and that is "being offended" (see below). You can't imagine how easily people got offended by my actions. I didn't know my behavior was offensive especially at this period of time in my life. Please see the last point under stressful situations and let me know if you feel the pain I was feeling.

The below is called "Offense" chart. These are the steps which takes place when a person allows offense to take charge in their life. It will take another book to give examples of mean, cruel and evil things people do to one another once offense is involved. I promise you, any person that allows the explosion of bitterness and/ or destruction take root in their heart; they are really sleeping with Evil in his bed. See the steps on the next page:

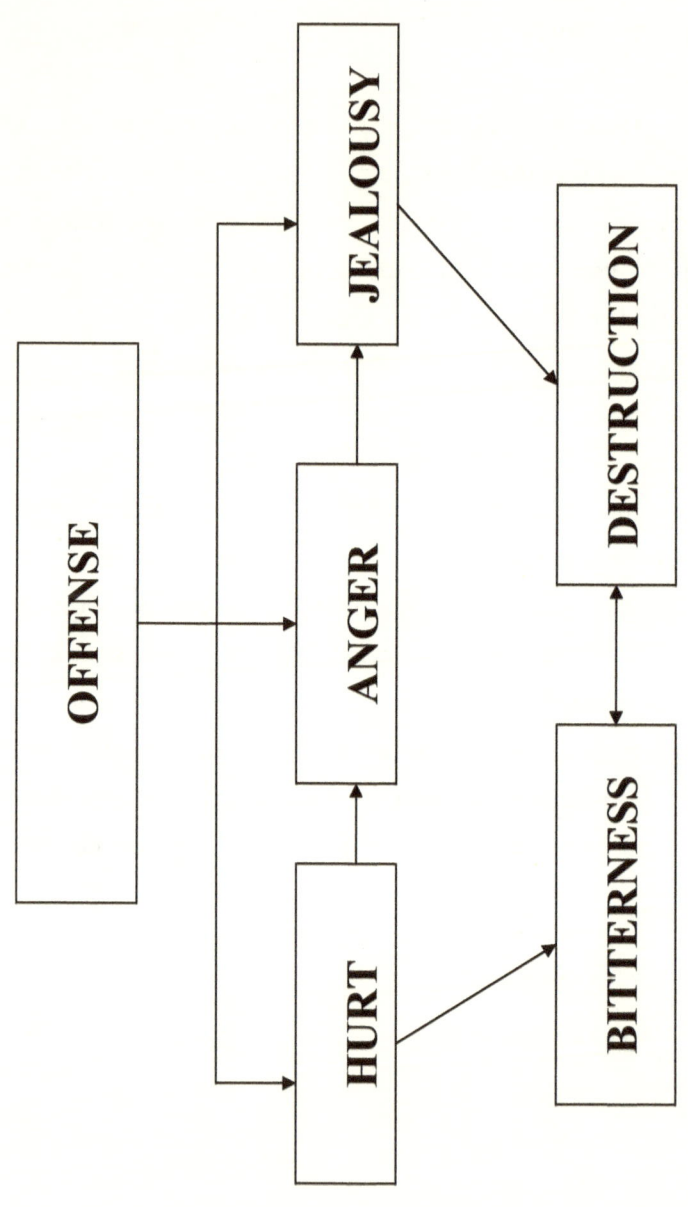

The Stressful Situations:

◆ I moved back home with my mom after living by myself for almost ten years. Her love is exceptional. She loved me even though we differ in religious beliefs.

◆ I offended Christian people that hurt me more than being sick. My whole understanding of priorities was out of order. The behavior caused anger toward me (Remember I was still dealing with MS).

◆ My mother had to pay for health insurance for me.

◆ I offended someone close too me. That caused a cold and angry treatment. (Remember I was still dealing with MS.)

◆ The tension of that action could have almost killed me by itself.

Then *the worst attack that happed to me*: the same type of emotional hurt that I experienced with people was the same type of hurt I caused to someone else. For almost two months the treatment literally caused me to relapse.

Again, I caused someone pain and in return I got paid back (I Cor. 8:12).

If you don't believe in God and you know or have known people with multiple sclerosis, there is no way this book could have been written without divine intervention. I am writing with pain in my hands and body, but I felt compelled to write this book now.

Miracle Number One

The fact that you are reading this book is a miracle all by itself. I had been diagnosed with multiple sclerosis in 2002. I didn't accept that Deborah Lovell—a woman of faith, strength, and power—had this terrible disease. I just chose to operate in faith and believe it would go away because I knew the Almighty God would not allow this to happen to me.

What a big mistake I made. You see, there was a lot of luggage that I was carrying besides multiple sclerosis. First of all, I slipped away from the word of God. Although I am a Christian and even went to ministry school, that didn't mean there weren't issues that needed to be addressed in my life.

I was so far gone I believed that my faith would touch God's heart and He would use me as an example to show that His healing power is true. Now He is truth—wonderful and powerful. The real truth is God and no one tells or instructs Him on when and how He does miracles.

My health was at stake and all of my decisions could have killed me even if I wasn't dealing with MS. There were different talks about eating right and eliminating certain foods from your diet. Of course, my A-type personality went straight for what I heard and thought was right and made a decision to eliminate red meat, sugar, and dairy products (Hosea 4:6).

Now you must realize I was a woman who never took care of her body prior to MS. Can you imagine how devasting it was to not eat foods that I really needed to eat because I didn't research or get proper help from a doctor on any nutrimental eating habits? My weight estimation went from 145 to 115 within months. We estimate that because we didn't record my weight, but the assumption was there due to my dress size. I went from ten to six.

As you noticed, it has already been a miracle that I am in position to write this book. Now that's a miracle!

Miracle Number Two

I will give you some of my history of emotional drama that it is believed to have caused or prevented me from accepting my needed treatments for MS.

The only people who knew how badly I was hit spiritually, physically, and emotionally were my family. My mom literally came up to the state of Michigan and moved me back to Georgia. If she had not made a decision to get her grown daughter out of the state at that time, there is no doubt in my mind I would have died. (Now that's a miracle.)

My life has been emotional from the time I was a young girl all the way up until I got hit with MS. The first blast was the way my father cursed me as a young girl when I was twelve. He got angry with me because he saw me sitting on one of my classmate's laps. This was a man who was not in my life as a father (That's another story. Let's stay with this part for now.)

I was in a park in our old neighborhood in Brooklyn, New York. The park was large. It was cut off in sections. There was a kiddy park and then the large part that included the basketball and handball courts. It would probably round up to about ten long blocks. Now imagine that he cursed at me from the kiddy park through the big park and three additional blocks until I got home.

The incident alone caused me to become an emotional person toward any type of hurt people caused me. Also, I had unforgiveness in my heart toward my father from that time on (1973) until I got saved in 1993.

The next emotional incident happen when my daughter's dad and I broke up. I had been dating him for fifteen years; he broke my heart beyond repair. It took two years for me to laugh or smile and I lost over twenty-five pounds within a couple of weeks. Please note, I only dated my daughter's father; I was not married to him (I Cor. 6:13).

The last emotional episode (remember I was dealing with MS) was an overwhelming stack of issues. I offended some Christian folks and their treatment was hurtful. Again, you now know some of my emotional background. What has been the most unbelievable thing for me to finally see is that I put Christian folks before my family and myself.

My whole life was out of order from my family to my health and relationships.

My body being attacked with MS didn't flow as smoothly as it could have. It would have been easier if I hadn't been carrying so much emotional drama. For example, I didn't take medicine when I first found out that multiple sclerosis really attacked my body because I thought God saw that I was operating for Him, so all was well. Hopefully reading this book will guide you to read the Bible for yourself and you can personally know the character of God is nothing like how I have attempted to describe Him from my previous recorded actions.

Finally I was able to get a good look at myself and didn't like what I saw (remember I was still dealing with MS). Here I was, a woman of God who was used in miracles, healing, and the spread of the Gospel, yet I had no evidence that Jesus Christ was my Lord and savior by my behavior.

1. I had tunnel vision.
2. I was blinded by (spiritual) pride and didn't know it.
3. I rejected anyone who wasn't singing my song.
4. I was judgmental and critical.
5. I put people before God and family.
6. I selectively loved people.
7. I lost compassion for people.

Make no mistake, I got the same treatment I dished out to people, but I couldn't understand why until now. Seed →Time →Harvest (Genesis 8:22).

Lastly, I found out through this pain and experience that the reason I was so emotionally affected by behavior of hurt was all the old emotions were raised back up when I got hit with MS and moved away from the word of God (II Cor. 5:17).

For example, my desire was to have a father and whole family that loved one another. When I got saved (Romans 10:17) God healed all those emotional scars, but you must stay hooked up with God in order keep His blessings to continue pouring down on you. Now that's a miracle!

It is my hope that if you are reading this and have MS, you will please address any emotional issues you have in a non-confrontational manner, and if there is any un-forgiveness (Matt. 6:14-15), strife, or bitterness, it must be eliminated (Heb. 12:15).

My point, is that if you have been diagnosed with MS, you can have a calm, smooth process and drama-free experience with no emotional issues attached if they are addressed with support and a heart of compassion (Heb. 5:2).

The SPE Support Group

This support function is designed for all women and men. When I first started with this program, I thought it would be targeted more toward African American women, but MS is no respecter of persons. Multiple sclerosis is an ugly, disrespectful, uncooperative disease. Throughout history African American women and people of color haven't had access to healthy support systems, but even more needed is a system that will really help a connection without feeling isolated, embarrassed, or unwanted.

Spiritual

An example of identifying a person where they are spiritual not only relates to them being a member of a church or their relationship with God, but the process also helps identify where they are inside. For example, can you smile or laugh? Are you angry, sad, or in denial that MS has really attacked your body?

My experience in dealing with this after going through some of the hurt was I didn't like myself. I totally took all the blame for mistakes, not recognizing that MS hit my body for real. It wasn't my imagination and I wasn't in position to control a lot of my actions. Remember I was blinded by pride and couldn't see the destructive pattern.

<u>Emotional</u>

Any emotional issues that are stress to your body need to be identified and dealt with immediately. For example, you can't have any negative attitude toward people, family, friends, bosses, pastors, ministers, etc. There is no exception. Your walk, look, speech, and conversation can be hurtful to a person that you may not like. Your presence can speak for itself even if you don't say anything that is good or bad.

I was diagnosed with MS in 2002 and lived in denial for one year. My body broke down in 2003 and my mom literally had to come and pick me up from one state and move me in her Atlanta home. There is a lot of history associated with this, but I will give you a synopsis of the emotional symptoms, which are the following:

(1) Depression

(2) Low self-esteem

(3) Laziness

(4) Hurt

(5) No value

(6) Self-hatred

(7) Judgmental

(8) Angry

(9) No Compassion

(10) Un-forgiveness

Experiencing all of those hurts or actions can and will destroy you if they are not addressed in some fashion. For example, before one of the flare-ups that occurred in my body; this is what happened. One, I received a treatment that went great; two, my new exercise program was going well; and three, my spirit was lifted up with a new hairdo.

My body literally broke down when I went out with a friend and saw someone from my past. The symptoms in my body were all the ten I listed, and they hit me at once. You can't imagine someone in that type of position. I remember saying to myself, *God, why did you allow that pain to occur in my life?* If you know anything about God, you know He is good all the time. We get ourselves in positions and then wonder why He didn't help. God doesn't violate your choices, whatever they may be.

Physical

It is very important to get exercise. I personally never paid any attention to the health of my body, and there is a very heavy price for that. A routine needs to be developed and committed to. This is something you have to be disciplined about. It is my belief that I will master an exercise routine.

Second Stage of Multiple Sclerosis

I have been diagnosed with remitting-relapsing MS. In 2003, all my symptoms appeared to indicate secondary progressive MS. I was home for a few weeks before I went right back in the hospital. The systems were: (1) loss of memory, (2) incomprehensive communication, (3) judgmental attitude, (4) unrealistic wants, (5) weakness in my body, (6) hurting those closest to me, (7) denial of the disease, (8) low self-esteem, (9) lack of trust, (10) looking toward people for my strength, (11) extreme vulnerability, and (12) inability to stop talking, etc.

Please remember I was a woman that who operated with a lot of pride (Proverbs 8:13). A person in that mindset doesn't realize what he or she is doing. In my experience it has been noted you become blind. This type of pride usually occurs in people who have A-type personalities and neglect family. Other people and job positions are their highlights, but not humbling (Matt. 8:4) yourself becomes very dangerous. Of course, a person operating in pride thinks they are humble. Here are some dangerous things you need to recognize if you are operating in pride: One, no one can do your work; two, you want to be involved in everything; and three, it is more important that you help everyone, etc.

Some of the things that helped me get on track were the following:

1. A faithful family and many friends from my church and a previous job shared and showed their love and support. More than thirty people (family, friends, and people from my church fellowship) showed their love and support, and for one year God had twelve people surround me and seven people call me every day. (Now that's a miracle.)

2. The Shepherd Center in Atlanta Georgia took me under its wing.

3. The medication taken slowed up the exacerbation attacks.

4. Bible scriptures and the experience of kindness (Psalms 23, Matt. 22:37, I John to 3

John, and Isa. 41:10) developed my heart at an even higher level of love than before MS.

5. Regaining a purpose to live and love again by helping others with MS.

6. Laughing and smiling sincerely from my heart and not for appearances sakes

7. The birth of my granddaughter was more joy than life. I felt like God gave me another opportunity to love my daughter as a baby again.

Although I am in a position to write this book, it has really taken me all the three years that I have been diagnosis to accept that my body is really being attacked by a disease.

My experience with MS has allowed me to see that people who don't have the disease can also exhibit the behavior associated with MS. For example, it was incredible to see how many people were judgmental (Luke 6:37) and critical. The sad point about that is I was just like them. It was only when hit with the terrible disease that I was able to see how very low I was and my actions displayed very few examples of Christ like behavior toward certain people.

Let me explain here that I was a woman born and raised in New York City and a real work alcoholic with no time and really had know idea a person could know God. The idea about walking in real love, or agape love, (God's type of love) was almost unbelievable. It was only after I went to a full Gospel church that I was able to see another type of life was prepared for me.

Can you believe I lived a sinful life, yet after God cleaned me up it seemed that I started treating people as if I was better than them? Remember we all sin and make mistakes, but after you know the real truth and allow it to change you, it is really hard to live a sinful life (Rom. 3:23). I now understand that God's grace has to be on you for you to not permanently live a sinful life.

Please believe me, it took multiple sclerosis for me to see all the scars that I hadn't healed from and the new scars I was causing my family and friends. Do you know hurting people will hurt and or damage other people?

The stage I am being treated for at this point is relapsing MS. It is a stage that I believe eventually will be without systems. That's because it is understood my body needs to be taken care of with the right medications and help from professionals, and my faith can continue, and it too can be an example of how wisdom was used in my healing process.

Family Matters

It is only after I fell down spiritually, physically, and emotionally that I was able to see how beautiful my family was. When you are in a down position, you can see all those hidden things that no one else sees because everyone is standing up.

My mom is an incredible person; she has the abilities of a nurse, a cook, a great-grandmother, a grandmother, and a mom. My sister and my daughter are such sweethearts. I asked the Lord why they are so kind and gentle and it seems like that those characteristics take a lot of work for me to flow like that (smile).

The answer was simple: I was hurt in two major instances in my past and the moment someone hurt my feelings, it made me close up. Again, through my teachings at church, it was great, and you know God can fix your broken heart. It's up to you as an individual to completely walk in that teaching. I must say an attack that hurts you spiritually, emotionally, and physically is designed to kill you.

Again, I am so grateful to God for my family. If another family member would have been hit with a disease like MS, it is hard to say if my actions would have been as compassionate as my family members. Thank God for the compassion (I John 3:17) in my heart for those with MS has allowed me to fight, love, and educate as many people as possible.

My family is one of the main reasons I can write this book. It would be impossible for me to share love and compassion about my faith had I had the same type of judgmental and condemning attitude before being attacked with MS.

The compassion and thanksgiving I have with my God and family would not have happened prior to MS. It is not a good thing, but my experience will help millions of other people; now that's a miracle.

As stated at the beginning of this book, listed on the following pages are questionnaires for you to answer to determine if you have MS or are causing symptoms of MS from an emotional standpoint. Note: I am not a medical doctor or expert on MS; my opinions are based on experience in my body from MS. See which questionnaire suits you. For example, there is one questionnaire for people who have MS, another for minorities (in New York City), and yet another for Christian folks who believe in the full gospel of the Bible.

I hope you have benefited from my experience and it is a help and blessing.

MULTIPLE SCLEROSIS

Or

MUTIPLE SCARS

(Exod. 15:26)

The purpose of this questionnaire is to help you immediately identify where you are in this disease. Please don't make the same mistake I did by denying you have multiple sclerosis. For one year I tried to continue ignoring the systems and could have died.

I thought because of my faith that a mighty miracle was going to happen and I was going to be an example for God to use. Now notice the spirit of pride and no wisdom. Please take the medicine.

If you are working in a highly stressful job, is it healthy and beneficial to leave? I can almost guarantee that your emotions are unstable—almost uncontrollable. That no one can understand unless they are dealing with MS.

Do you find yourself trying harder for others to see you are in control and hoping they like you more because you are emotional vulnerable? The questionnaires relate to my own breakdown. They are designed for the multiple sclerosis patients, minority patients, and Christian patients.

For the MS patient:

1. Are you in denial about MS?

2. Do you take medication or decide not to?

3. Can you still do your job if you work?

4. What emotions have changed since you been diagnosed?

5. Is there a desire to please people like never before?

For the family:

1. Did you investigate the symptoms of MS?

2. Have you spoken to a neurologist who specializes in MS?

3. Is there a support group or affiliation that can assist you?

4. How many family members are participating in helping?

5. Do you know how important it is to have those diagnosed with MS to be, spiritually, emotionally, and physically nurtured?

MUTIPLE SCLEROSIS

Or

MUTIPLE SCARS

(Matt. 7:1-6)

Minorities can relate to these questions, but I am sharing my hurt as an African American Woman. Multiple sclerosis is an ugly disease, and if you have no experience with it, you can't relate in any form or fashion to how it affects a person.

We are at a point in time that you must recognize the end is coming. Whether you believe in God or not, something is really wrong in today's world. That I believe we all can agree on. Listed below are questions geared toward minorities.

I don't need to go into history, but MS is too hard for people to deal with, and having the hurts that come along with being treated wrongly can cause total destruction within a person diagnosed with MS.

For the minority patient:

My background is some what mixed out of four grandparents; two of my grandparents were from Barbados, one was from Jamaica, and one was African American. When my grandmother from Barbados passed away, that destroyed the communication in that entire part of the family. We were closet to my African American folks. Let me tell you it is sad the way we treat each other. I mean it's hard enough with the regular prejudices, and when blacks from other countries are prejudiced against their American brothers and sisters, this only makes the evil one of this world (John 10:10), who wanted the separation, succeed. Can you imagine dealing with MS and prejudices within your own race of people?

For the minority patient:

1. Do you know someone who has multiple sclerosis?

2. Are from America or another country?

3. How do you treat your brothers and sisters?

4. Do interact with or make an attempt to reach out to others?

5. Did you hear the myth that African American women don't like woman from other countries?

MUTIPLE SCLEROSIS

Or

MUTIPLE SCARS

(Luke 10:30-34)

Please, before you start reading, assuming you are a Christian, ask this question to God: simply say Father, am I going to heaven? You may think that is not something that needs asking. Of course, if you are a man or woman of God and have been in the ministry for such a long time, living prosperous, and all is good, you may even be doing your ministry assignment. However, if you purposely treated anyone of God's children in an ugly way (I John 3:15) and caused their souls to go to hell, I can guarantee, you are not going to heaven according to the Word of God (Matthew 7:22-23) without repentance (I John 1:9).

Everyone who claims to be a believer in the Lord must have a personal relationship with him. I would have never have thought my actions were religious until I got around nonbelievers. There was no Agape love shown on my behalf. Here I was, a ministry school graduate used mightily for God, yet my experience didn't stop my judgmental behavior.

For the Christian patient:

1. Are you really operating in the love of God toward your brothers and Sisters in Christ? (1 Cor. 13:1-15)

2. Have you poisoned other people toward someone who offended you?

3. Do you have God in the right place? (Matt. 6:33)

4. How would you share love with someone you don't like?

5. Did you ask God if you were going to heaven? What did he say?

6. Can you honestly say your behavior toward your brothers and sisters who are less fortunate than you makes them see you as an example?

I don't take for granted that you have received Jesus Christ as your Lord and Savior. It is very simple to receive Jesus Christ as Lord and Savior.

This is what you do. Simply say this prayer:

Dear Jesus,

I believe that you died for me and that you rose again on the third day. I Confess to you that I am a sinner and that I need your love and forgiveness.

Come onto my life, forgive my sins, and give me eternal life. I confess to You now as my Lord. Thank you for my salvation!

It is just that simple to be Saved; now it takes studying the word of God (the Bible), attending church, and learning how to be like Jesus. Now that will take your life, but let's take it one step at a time. God bless!

It is a matter of urgency that you find a church that ministers the word of God from the Bible. God's word is so true. Your life will change through my own experience. Get a bible that you can read and comprehend; start reading The New Testament—first the book of John.

Read a powerful prayer out of the Bible and put your name in it (Eph. 1:17-23).

If you have access to the Internet, log on to some of the networks such as www.mhmin.org. www. creflodollarmin.org, and www.joycemyers.org each of these sites has great information on prayer, which is one of the most important steps in being a Christian who loves God and understanding true Christian life. It is my prayer that after you do These steps you will be able to identify a church home in Jesus's name!

It is my hope if people can love like this:

Matt.22:37 Jesus said unto him, Thou shalt love the Lord thy God with all thy heart, and with all thy soul, and with all thy mind.

It is my sincere desire that you were blessed by the writing of this book. I can honestly say it has made me a free woman for God to use as he so pleases. PRAISE GOD!

Deborah Lynn Lovell

(Multiple Sclerosis 2002-2007)

404-680-1751

Multiple Sclerosis is a disease had I personally not come in contact with it, I would never have understood the anger, neglect, hurt and pain people experience with that disease.

My overall life experience is very diverse, Health Care, Hospice and a Patent & Trademark law firm in New York City and now a graduate of ministry school. My love for people allowed me to enjoy my jobs.

The below are steps that took on it's own meaning in my life that will hopefully help others to never give-up.

Vita Journa/Aug-2007.............................Trivita
                www.trivita.com
                (Deborah's comment about the B-12 Sublingual)

(2004-2007)
SPE System................................E-Mail Buddies
(Spiritual, Physical and Emotional)

Games: The 4Cs (Compassionate, Considerate,
                        Consistent and Committed)
            The Questions and The Tidbits

(2006-2007)
CURE..................................Research Project
        www.accleratedcure.org

(2006-2007)
Educational Ambassador................Multiple Sclerosis
        www.msaa.com   Association of America

(2005-2007)
Book Published............................No More MS

(2005)
Article Written on Deborah............Wellness A State
By **Karen Neff, LMT ma#0031617**   of Mind
        kfneff@comcast.net